HOW TO BE A FITNESS BADASS

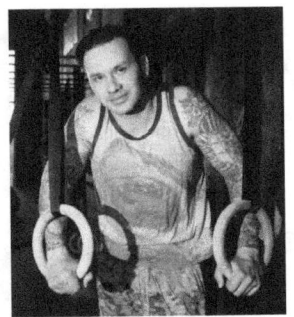

Cross Training For Elite Athletes
With A champion's Mentality

BY

JACOB C. HOWELL

ACKKNOWLEDGMENTS

SPECIAL THANKS TO MY FAMILY, my parents, brothers, and sister, and all those who have supported my efforts as I have pursued my dreams.

Also to Coach Jeff "Mad Dog" Madden, University of Texas Strength and Conditioning.
Coach 'Pete' and Rene Pena with the St. Louis Cardinals (MLB) Organization.
Coaches D. Maib and Bennie Wylie Strength and Conditioning Coaches
Coach David Deets, the guy that introduced me to chase this career.
Coaches Todd Stroud and Jon Jost at Florida State University that allowed me the first opportunity to coach with them at a college level with the Strength and Conditioning program.
Coach Tom Schubert UTPA Basketball who allowed me to handle the strength and conditioning program with his players when that led us to win our independent championship.
Coach Stan Bonewitz, Athletic Director, Concordia University at Austin.
I will always keep in mind, "Slow and steady wins the race" Judges 16:28

INTRODUCTION

My first exercise equipment given to me was not a bench or a pair of dumb bells, but a rake and wheel barrel. As crazy I thought my dad was, it taught me hard work, pride, dedication and discipline. Which has led me to the person I am today. Those same traits have led me to train elite athletes and becoming a fitness world champion and author on fitness. One of the main problems in today's world is everyone wants the overnight success, no pain, no struggle; just given. The problem with that is the struggle and pain through life experiences that make you stronger and a better person are omitted. Elite Fitness or becoming a fitness badass will be earned not given. The most common example is the popular New Year's resolutions **"lose weight and look better & healthier"**. The problem is, every year you might be saying the same thing. Everyone wants the overnight success. "If you're tired of the same old routine, it's time you challenge your fitness to a whole new level. Included will be the blue print to your self-confidence and fitness success. Through my years of experiences I trained myself and elite athletes. The fastest and most efficient way to elite fitness or becoming a fitness badass is training like an "elite athlete".   This 6 week exercise program uses cross training and strength & conditioning designed to cut body fat, build muscle, and improve your overall body fitness.

I hope you take the information in this book to heart. I have placed a lot of my years and studies to help you become the 'best you that you can be'. Dreams can come true. It's never too late to get fit. There were too many obstacles that I had overcome in my growing years; I knew I could change myself into a person I wanted to be. You might have the same thoughts. I made a plan, followed it, focused, and became determined to stick with it. Within four months I lost close to sixty pounds. I followed the fitness and meal plan I had researched. I was enjoying what I was accomplishing. I even entered fitness and sports modeling competitions. My hard work and dedication has led me to win such titles the **Natural Sports Fitness National and World Championship and National Sports Model Physique Champion**. My qualifications now include: Master's Degree Bachelor's Degree, Certified Personal Trainer, SCCC- CSCCA Certified Strength and Conditioning, Certified College & Professional Strength and Conditioning, Elite Nike SPARQ Trainer, and Certified Speed Coach. My thirst for knowledge to be the best has led me to have trained elite athletes by being on the Strength staff for the World Champion St. Louis Cardinals, Florida State, Concordia University and the University of Texas. I haven't even hit forty yet. The road has had some bumps but has given me great opportunities. God has blessed me with these great experiences. Nothing great will come easy, you're gonna have to ask yourself, "Do you want it?" It's all up to you. Get on board and follow your dreams. Be the fitness badass you want to be! Remember, you are one of the GREATEST MACHINES ever created.

HOW TO BECOME A FITNESS BADASS

One's health condition is probably the highest priority one should consider evaluating. There are three areas when one looks as our health; mind, emotional, and physical state. All three are as important; not one is more important than the other. Like the laws of physics and nature, balance is the key. Imbalance can deter improper function and thus there is lack of harmonious function within the human body. There is a fourth area which is just as important but I will not cover, that is personal and up to the individual; the spiritual.

The mind is the controller and the decision maker of the body. It is vital that one understands the power of the mind. If one does not care about the mind, it will affect one's life tremendously. Information we put into it and or ignore will affect our decisions whether we want to admit it or not. We learn by visual, by hearing, and by experiencing. The latter is very important and the one less placed attention to. For example, one learns that people should not do drugs and drive, but everyday individuals ignore facts , thus ignoring what they know is true. Therefore, one must understand that we must learn to not only train and educate the mind but once it has recorded the information, we need to learn to listen when it recalls the information then reminds us what to do with the information. Unfortunately, we have a free will that might to go against a warning. We will cover this later in the book.

Secondly, our emotions also play a huge role in our balance with our body. As humans, we can be very emotional; gender is equal in emotions but some individuals are more emotional than others. Emotions are good and very healthy, however, we also need to learn to keep a balance and control them to a degree. Love, insecurity, hate, anger, ambition, aggressiveness, fear, and worry, are some of the emotions that can overpower the condition of a person. At times, the unbalance can lead to stress, nervousness, and even take an individual to acquire mental problems. All these emotions can be controlled what I feel plays an important strength in utilizing emotions to one's benefit. This strength is ATTITUDE! Believe or not, our attitude we take when confronting our daily lives is our attitude we counter with. I will cover four areas of attitude; optimism, pessimism, realism, and opportunism. Like the mind, we need to learn to listen to our emotions and learn to utilize which attitude we need to take. We must learn to utilize the energy our body outputs with emotion. They can lead to bad or good outcomes and even lead to life saving decisions. The same event can allow and individual to lead to needing to change to survive while on another individual can lead to suicide as an escape. The attitude applied can make the difference. We will discuss this to more detail later in the book.

Thirdly, the physical is the outer and more oblivious of the three. The package and the packaging usually is what we look at when 'buying' or 'choosing' a product. Even when we are born, we look for signs of health of the newborn by its physical package. Blood tests, X-rays, and sonar cannot prove or disprove mental or emotional health. Therefore, the physical is the carrier for the self. It is the only of the three areas that is tangible. Most of our lives, we look at the physical whether in ourselves or in others. For that reason, we are creatures that will focus more on the physical than the other two. But, a balance is needed for a healthy body; mind, emotion, and body.

The first question or concern one needs to ask is; are you satisfied or happy with your current state of yourself; mind, emotional state, and physical state. If you are, there is always room for improvement. If you are not or want to improve yourself, this book will help you. It is my intent, with this book and my personal experiences, to improve you and improve all three areas for a total healthy being. I cannot guarantee a 100% improvement. That is up to you. One, we need to understand that we are creatures that are determined by our actions and decisions. Generally, we cannot blame others for our actions. We need to realize that we are products of our daily decisions and actions. If we decide not to study, exercise, and eat unhealthy, our health will suffer. If we decide to hang around with vultures, we will become as one of them. If we decide to hang around with eagles, perhaps it might persuade us to try to become as an eagle and fly like one. To be a fitness badass we need to have the inner power, drive, discipline, and confidence to become the best individual we can be!

. Through history we have learned that all cultures have tried to find ways to improve the health of the mind, body, and emotions. The ancient Jews had laws on what foods were clean and unclean for our bodies. I have always been fascinated with the Greek statues and their search for the perfect physical structural human body showing a high level of fitness. The Greeks were really into the physical body and the philosophy of the mind (attitude). The Eastern civilizations were into emotional health and physical fitness. Have you ever wondered why the oriental monks would meditate while making a continuous hummmming sound? The hum was to exercise the Pituitary gland in the middle lower base of the brain. This gland controls the growth of the body but it also helps all the glands in the body. By humming, they felt it was vibrating and exercising the Pituitary gland. I cannot assure you it works, but they felt it did.

Talk about the importance of the human body working in harmony, it has 206 bones, 640 muscles, 13 glands, approximately 70 trillion cells, 12 organs, and 11 pints of blood that feed, oxidize, and clean each living cell. Wow, what a working machine. To know how the human body has achieved miraculous feats like under the four minute mile, high jumping over seven feet, leaping over twenty-nine feet, and sprints under ten seconds in the one-hundred meters are mind blogging. That is why I named my first book, "The Greatest Machine". The body you possess is the only body you are going to have. Realistically, it's up to you to take care of it. You're stuck with it. Many individuals don't believe in pre-maintenance, well maybe on their machines like the car, lawnmower, a/c, etc. they do. But the human body also needs a lot of maintenance and pre-maintenance. Human nature has taught us that until something breaks that is when we finally take action. Necessity is the MOTHER of invention or need for change. Until we become overweight, under-weight, weak, out of shape, blood pressure rises or drops, or ill, we get concerned about our diet and physical body. This leads me to why I focused on writing this book. I hope you will allow me to focus on your total health; mind, body, and emotions so you can be a fitness badass and conquer everyday's challenges and obstacles.

CHAPTER I.

THE BLUE PRINT

Stage One: The Plan and Self evaluation

1. Are you satisfied with your weight? Height is out of the question.
2. Are you exercising enough, not enough, or not at all?
3. Are you eating healthy? (be honest with yourself}
4. How's your self-esteem? (Do you like yourself)
5. Are you generally happy?
6. Do you have a stressful life?
7. Do you get enough rest and sleep?
8. Are bad habits interfering in your overall daily events?
9. Are you financially overloaded or unstable?
10. Does your lifestyle choice's prevent you from your progress?

If you answered the above questions truthfully, we are ready to start!

Imagine owning your favorite dream vehicle. (Perhaps a Ferrari, or a super nice Truck, or a SUV) If you want it to last and perform its best you would you use the best oil, tires, and preventive maintenance. You would probably check the air in the tires regularly and all fluids required. I'm sure you would not run it on bad roads or leave it exposed to bad environmental hazards either. I am sure you would try to protect it and take care of it as much as possible **IF YOU CARED!**

Remember that your body is the only one you will have even if you decide to add plastic, Botox, or silicone. If you can apply a higher priority on your body, or what the Bible refers to as God's temple, than what you would use on your dream car, your body would always be in a better condition than the average person takes care of it. We take our body for granted. One can paint, place nice stickers, or stripes on the vehicle, add a nice stereo, spray nice fragrances, polish the leather, and wax it the outer surfaces, but if one does not take care of the operational mechanical parts of the vehicle, it will only be in vain. Eventually the vehicle was not perform correctly and breakdown. Again, hope you get the picture. The human body will eventually breakdown too if not taken care of and provided with pre-maintenance.

FIRSTLY, what is it that you want to do with your body? Do you have a PLAN? As you do your self-evaluation you need to also do a mental picture a NEW YOU!! This might seem insignificant but it's a major step. It is the beginning and first baby step towards a new direction or plan. Don't take it lightly. I remember my dad telling me that when he was in Vietnam, every time he was sent on a dangerous mission in which he was going to be gone out behind enemy lines, he would go to the base exchange (BX) and buy a shirt, a watch, or a new music cassette tape and not open it from its package. He had realized he could not depend on long range goals like going home or being home. Those were unrealistic at the time. What was realistic was coming back a few weeks later and wearing the new shirt or listening to the new cassette. As soon as he returned from his mission, he would open the gift he had bought for himself. As small as they were, they kept him focused for an immediate reward. So will it be with your plan and small steps. Let's say your goal is to get into a size 6 dress. Go buy it and make it your goal. As a personal trainer, that is one of my priorities to my clients; setting goals are very important. This will be part of the emotional state that will contribute to the physical aspect. We will refer to it as ATTITUDE. It has to be positive and optimistic. It is a proven fact that positive and optimistic individuals are more successful than their counterparts --- the negative and pessimists of the world. They tend to give up and lose faith regularly. Common sense verifies the last statement. Unfortunately we cannot go buy an attitude; we have to convince ourselves of getting one. It's the first battle within the mind. WE will discuss with more detail later in this book. If you cannot convince yourself, you will not succeed. Perhaps it may seem hard but one has to confront and jump head-first and commit yourself otherwise you become your greatest enemy; It is YOUR battle.

SECONDLY, you must plan the **TIME**. As we all know, time is precious. We catch ourselves trying to find time to do everything we need to do. A time block must be set. Flexibility will be needed at times, but a set time block needs to be set in semi-stone. You immediate loved must also learn that set time is important. Only attitude is the biggest deterrent to time for your new change. Try to set aside one hour. Yep, one hour, that will be all you need. One hour per day for at least four-five days of the week. Look at it as an investment that might prolong your life and give you an overall healthier lifestyle. Don't allow guilt or negative feelings push you away from your plan or dream. Keep focused. Remember, the largest tree in the forest started off as a tiny seed. Your total health will be your ultimate reward. I remember when I was getting my lifeguard license as a teenager, I asked my dad why was the training and test to be a lifeguard so difficult. He responded by telling me that an unprepared weakling cannot save a desperate individual. A well rounded healthy parent will be a better parent and ultimately prepared better for their responsibilities required. Unhealthy parents will be at times unresponsive, too tired, irritable, too stressed-out, or ill to be there for their children. And as we all know, now days, they are a handful. Probably every world champion in an athletic event has made found the time in the early hours of the day. They get up and put forth their effort just to train the body, emotions, and mind to place their goal as their highest priority! In a way, it again proves that self-discipline in very important.
THIRDLY, find a place where you will do the activities/exercises. It can be a gym, a park, or even at your own home. Pick a place where you will not be distracted from your focus. **Advise**: <u>If you pick a place where you will be easily distracted, it will eventually make it harder for you to focus and achieve your goals and dreams.</u> Example; if you take your child with you, naturally one eye will be on your goal and the other on your child. It is normal but realistically a deterrent. So, it's up to you. Know your tolerance and what you can or cannot handle.

CHAPTER II

THE METAMORPHIS

(BECOMING THE NEW YOU)

Discipline is one of the greatest sources of success. It can either make you or break you. The most notorious convicts and worst individuals can be broken in prison or in the military. If you ever visit a prison or a basic military training base, you can see individuals who were 'un-trainable' on the outside. In the structured environment, they follow orders like kinder-garden kids. Spoiled kids that never did any chores at home find themselves making their bunk beds that pass inspection, fold their military clothes, and even sweep and mop their living quarters without questioning their training instructors. You ought to see how they march in line and stay in line in the cafeteria and the first words out of their mouths usually start with "Sir, yes sir". The same applies to most prisoners. Of course there will be misfits that will take more time to break, but EVERYONE has a breaking point. I recall my high school coaches and how they tried to teach us that it was important we placed the training they were giving us was for our own good. If I could turn back the clock, I should have listened. I know I would have done better than what I did. Being young and immature is not a good mix. Do I have regrets? Of course I do. Thank God I have matured to understand and now try help my students not commit the errors many young athletes do. This book cannot discipline you. It will only require that YOU self-discipline yourself. I constantly find myself encouraging my athletes to work harder. This is actually the best and the hardest kind of discipline – **self discipline!**

I recall my junior high and high school days as an athlete and student. Do I have regrets? Of course I do! "If only I could have done this instead of that and if I could have done that instead of this." Sound familiar? When I played college basketball I was more mature but still not as self-disciplined as I should have. I look back and wished I could have pushed myself harder and maybe even taken constructive criticism better. I learned that procrastination was a monster. I have learned that TOMORROW never comes or gets here. When I thought I got to tomorrow, another tomorrow was there just as sure as yesterday. One has to learn to live for the moment and for the day; live for TODAY. Like the Latin motto; "Carpe Diem" which means "Seize the day". In short, self-discipline is for NOW, not yesterday or for tomorrow.

FOCUS is also an important part of self-discipline. Tiger Woods did not go practice football or basketball during his time off. Cam Newton did not go practice tennis when he had spare time. Thomas Edison did not read poetry in the library. I think you get the picture. Tiger focused on golf, Newton focused on football, and Edison focused on science. A master athlete, scientist, medical doctor, or whatever profession, must focus to be the best at what they dream to be. This very facet is important to a satisfactory degree for you to acquire your goals. If you live as if there was no tomorrow or this was your last chance to get your desire, your drive and attitude would surge to a superior level. But as I stated before, we take life and time for granted and don't take the opportunities at times placed at or feet!

I recall a short anecdote about a optimist, a pessimist, and a realist. They were debating over the old comparison of life utilizing a half-full glass of wine. The 'optimist' tried to convince the others how positive life can be despite half of life can be full of problems but that there was so much to be blessed with. The 'pessimist' tried to convince the others that life was so hard and full of problems despite good things that can happen. The 'realist' then took his side and tried to convince them that realistically we need to embrace both the good and the bad and learn to cope with both. Once the debate was over, they went back to the half-filled glass of wine and noticed it was empty. They were in wonder and asked what had happened to the wine. A gentleman stood up and said, "While you guys were arguing over your point of view for life, I drank the wine," answered the 'opportunist'. Sometimes we got do just that, embrace the opportunities that are placed in front of us. Here is an opportunity for you to change your total health and take your fitness to the next level. Do you have the self-discipline, time, and drive? Yesterday is gone, tomorrow might not get here, will you take advantage of today or the NOW?

I hope you realize I have probably taught you nothing yet. I hope you realize you already knew what I have covered thus far. The "will you do it?" and the "will to do it" are separated by your own self-discipline.

CHAPTER III.

GOING THROUGH THE FIRE
(OVERCOMING ADVERSITY)

I will the first to warn you that it will not be easy. There will be far too many obstacles that will try to delay or stop you from achieving your goals and dream. Everyone has their personal battles unknown only to them. There will logical and illogical thoughts, statements, and situations that will either try to convince you or actually stop you from going forward in your attaining your dream. Did I have that? I would be lying if I did not admit that I was attacked from all angles. I probably fell as many times as Thomas Edison burned light bulbs as he finally perfected the bulb that finally worked.

There were dark days in my life I usually I hate to discuss as you probably have yourselves. At an early age in my life, my parents got divorced. I grew up at times moving around and sharing home life styles. At times I got caught in the middle of family and divorce problems. There were days I wished I would not have been born. Love kept me afloat. At a very young age I learned to survive and appreciate the 'now'. I wanted to achieve and be somebody. To succeed in whether grades or games filled the void left in my heart due to the pain in my parents' divorce. As I grew and became a middle school student, I started to be bullied by older students. I was bullied verbally, emotionally, and physically. My dad took me and one of his friends that taught me boxing and karate. He also enrolled me in a fitness gym so I could develop my strength and confidence. I was tall and lanky full of dreams but the bullies kept interfering with my dreams. I never interfered with anybodies much less theirs. In fact, I always tried to stand up for younger kids that were being bullied by my peers. This time no one stood up for me because my peers feared the older and bigger bullies that bullied me. I look back at some of those jocks or wanna-be tough guys. Have you ever wondered why wolves and cowards hang around in packs?

I practiced boxing and karate 'fighting' for months until I was confident enough to defend myself. Bullying got complex because now I was fighting back. Physically, I grew and was able to defend myself pretty well. Unfortunately, the bullying continued but this time I was attacked by numbers because I could handle a one on one scenario. Was it demoralizing? You bet it was! Those days were so dark. What kept me going forward were my parent's love and my athletic ability. The bullying continued into my high school years. Some persons and coaches would rather turn a blind eye than discipline those who bullied me. It got to the point that my dad took me to another school district where he was now working. The bullying did not stop. The same bulls would go to where I then played just to distract my performance. I was recognized in football and basketball as All-District, All-Valley, and All-Area. I was even offered Division I opportunities in football in California, New Mexico and Texas universities. It was confusing to me how to handle coming from a small high school and going to a Division I college. Had I accepted I would have gotten the last laugh? My lack of self-confidence held me back. I enrolled in college. Affected by dark days in my life plus not controlling my self-discipline and anger. Partying became frequent as a way to handle my problems. I went into depression and could not function as well in college. I could have given up in life. My support circle was minimal. I was down to my parents and God. The most negative thoughts became part of my every day. I recall one day one of my professors took me outside his classroom and told me that I was not college material and for me to look for some alternative means of supporting myself. I was weak in advanced college math. One of my professors took me out into the hall. He told me to drop his class and consider dropping out of college. At this point he knocked the air out and my attitude changed that attending college was no longer my priority. That day was an eye opener. As painful as it was I knew I had to do something with my life. I re-evaluated myself. I prayed. I talked to my dad to help me.

It took months for me to pick myself up. I actually dropped out of college. I did not want to be idle with my life. At one point, I wanted to be an engineer. I even went and talked to the Navy recruiter. I was about to sign. He had painted a beautiful picture of me doing so great in the Navy. He even showed me a video where the Navy guys were playing basketball on the deck of the huge ship. My parents did not give up on me. The day the Navy recruiters showed up to pick me up the door was respectfully slammed in their face. My parents knew it would have been for the wrong reasons; to escape reality and try to run from my problems instead of confronting them. They knew better. I picked myself up and took a chance and applied at a college and walked on to the basketball team. I got my grades up, re-did my college plan, focused on my skills and made the team. I realized that I was the solution to my life's problems. I had allowed things I could not control drive me away from my expectations and my realistic abilities. I had no control of my parent's divorce. I had allowed those who had hateful bullying ways push me away from the school I loved. I had allowed bad study habits and bad choices to intrude into my mental state. I found the guilty one. It was me. I had listened more to the negative people in my life than those who tried to help me. I saw myself as a victim rather than a winner. In my lowest points in my life, there were lessons to learn. I had not taken the opportunities to learn from my down falls. But now I was learning and no longer blamed myself. My new coaches at my new high school kept telling me to keep my head up and not to give up. They saw my potential but I saw my wounds. They tried to heal them but I only licked them. Yes, I know there will be adversary and obstacles. I recall my dad's stories how he had to overcome fear during combat and flying over enemy lines. He had to overcome PTSD and Agent Orange that affected his heart condition. He is disabled but continues to enjoy life. So, as you have learned before, it's not how many times you fall, it's getting up that matters. You have to learn as I did, sometimes no one might want to pick you up or be there to pick you up, you must learn to **PICK YOURSELF UP** that matters. There will always be 'haters' and individuals that will try to deter and hold you back. Kiss them good-bye. You don't need negative individuals in your life.

You will run into injuries and health issues that might only slow you down or make you change roads, but you must learn to make adjustments and keep focused on the path for self-preservation and be the best you were made to be. I felt I was at a breaking point but I had to use it as a lesson rather than a defeat. I remember reading once that we were all born because we had already been a winner when we were that ONE sperm to get through the mad race to get to be the one to enter the egg awaiting as we battled and became the victor and became a human body. We were not made to be losers. We become a product of our attitudes, actions, and decisions. We at times don't realize what we can do with ourselves. We spend too much time paying attention to no-gooders and individuals that wish us bad. Whether envy, hate, or just ill will, it will always exist. How we learn to handle it will determine our success or failures. In a nut shell, it's up to us and only us to make oneself the best we can be.

I have seen individuals who have been crippled or disfigured to accidents or crime yet overcome those fierce obstacles and still succeed. I admire those individuals and highly respect them. I refuse to belittle others. I refuse to judge others. I refuse to hold anyone from trying to attain their dreams. I have made that part of my mission. I will always encourage, support, and assist in helping others seek betterment. This is another reason for being honest and forthcoming in this book. I want all to know that we need to do the same for other – especially our youth.

My self-confidence and ability to overcome obstacles made me that much stronger and will to defy the odds. I got to finish my education and get my degree in Engineering. Well, not really, I was told I could not be an engineer ---- well, I became an Engineer of the Greatest Machine, the Human Body; **Kinesiology** with certification in Exercise Physiology. Few years later I attained my Master's degree and even when I was discouraged by my college counselor. It made me even more determined to defy the norm! I volunteered my time to help with the basketball program at Oklahoma State University. Coach Eddie Sutton saw and appreciated the enthusiasm for coaching. It was not an over-night success but rather a low process of steps in finally reaching my dreams and goal. He gave me the opportunity that opened the doors at Florida State as Strength and Conditioning coach. That opened a door to coach at the University of Texas with the strength and conditioning department under Coach Jeff Madden. That opened the door to get a similar position with the professional baseball team St. Louis Cardinals in which I got the opportunity to train world class and world champion athletes. In 2010 I competed in various body building contests. I placed in a couple. Then I won the state championship for the state of Texas in Sports Fitness and Sports Modeling. I was invited to the world competition to be held in Hollywood California. I asked my dad If he would go with me. His first reaction was not too positive. He felt I didn't stand a chance and knew I would be discouraged but he agreed to go with me. My prayers and dream were answered. I became a World Champion in my division at the INBA National Natural Fitness competition event. My first thoughts were, if all the 'jocks' who bullied me could see me now. I held my trophy in their honor. It was them who made me fight back and become what none of them could ever earn or take away. If they only knew **they** helped me become what I have accomplished. It was their negativity and evil wishes that finally drove me to success. It was taking their lemons to make my great lemonade. None of them ever played college ball much less coach at a collegiate or professional level. I sometimes feel or hear their negative and childish language, but I remind myself where that took me and I thank God and all those who believed in me, but ultimately it had to take me to believe in me! If you have had such negativity poured on you, take it as fuel to reach your goal.

Learn to wear Teflon skin and just allow the negativity thrown at you to slide off. Learn to know what you can control and what you cannot control. Learn to pick yourself up when you are down. You were the winning sperm. God does not make losers. Learn to find the inner strength to overcome the **HATERS** who want to keep you down. Learn to seek a positive comfort zone. Learn to seek a positive support system. Learn to accept yourself. Learn to love yourself. Learn that the better individual you are the more you can help better others. Learn to give, not take. Learn to listen, not just talk. Learn to live as if there was no tomorrow. Learn to walk in other's shoes. Learn not to judge. Finally, don't take life for granted; find your purpose in your life and learn to **"RISE ABOVE ALL"**.

Logic sometimes is hard to really understand. Remember when we would see a small angel on one shoulder and a small devilish character on the other shoulder? Both try to convince the individual with convincing statements. They were both great debaters and had good solid answers whether right or wrong. This is another scenario every individual will have to confront as an over-comer. Suave statements like "Do you really need this pain just to lose a few pounds, no one really cares". Or, how about, "Enjoy being who you are, just eat a little less next time, that will work". How about, "You had your youth, you need to take it easy and everybody loves you the way you are anyway".

This will be the part you must learn to beat. It's being able to beat yourself; the inner you. We all have a smart side and a foolish side. We all have a good side and a bad side. I recall a story I heard once from a speaker regarding an old American Indian tale regarding an old grandpa teaching his young grandson about inner strength. He told his grandson that in all of us live two wolves; one bad and one good. That one wolf gets its strength from being evil, bad, lying, greedy, and all things that are not good. The other wolf that lives within us is one of love, compassion, honesty, giving, and all the good things. The grandpa continued to tell his grandson that they do battle every day. When the young grandson asked his wise grandpa who would win, the grandpa answered, "which ever you feed, wins". This is the true answer in character building. The decision you make will uncover your real strength and courage you need. It won't be easy. Have you ever noticed that the conscience never lies or is wrong? The conscience will clear up right from wrong while the dark side will try to convince you that doing the wrong thing is justifiable.

We'll call the conscience the Right side and we'll call the devilish side, the Left side. Let the debate start.

Left side, "It's too expensive, will take too much time, will keep you away from things you need to do, and besides, your love handles are customized to your body".

Right side, "Think of your health and self-esteem. Think of how you total body and your muscle tone will benefit. Your loved ones will have to adjust to your personal needed time. Your health is important on the long run."

Left side, "What? What if you hurt yourself doing exercises? You don't have the time or energy for fantasies. You need to understand that you need to be accepted the way you look and how you are. If someone really needs you, it shouldn't matter how you look. Your appearance doesn't matter anymore. You are not in high school anymore so just learn to live as you are.

Right side, "Think of your health and there is nothing wrong with getting on a rigid diet, vigorous exercise program, and work on your self-esteem. Become a fitness badass so it can take you to the level you need to be in. It's going to take some sacrifice and dedication; all worth it!

Left side, "That's right, you only live once, so take it easy, not worth the time and pain."

Right side, "Make your move, let's see how smart you are!"

After that scenario and self-debate, what seems logical to you? You know Mr. Right is correct! Obstacles will arise from every direction and you need to be flexible, but you must not give up. There will be bumps, delays, and at times adjustments, but don't CANCEL your goal or dream.

STORY OF THE BUTTERFLY

I remember my dad telling me the story of a man once walking home. As he walked through the path he noticed a cocoon half open and a butterfly struggling to get out from the cocoon casing. He passed on and then thought that it might die while it struggled to get out. He quickly returned to the small branch where the cocoon was. The butterfly was almost half out but still struggling. The man decided to use his knife and cut open the cocoon and allow the struggling butterfly to come out easier and quicker. He felt he had done a good deed and saved the butterfly by cutting the cocoon and prevent pain and un-necessary struggle by the new transformation of the worn into a beautiful butterfly. The following day he took the same path. As he approached the branch where he had performed the good deed, he found the now empty cocoon. He smiled and felt so relieved that the butterfly had survived the struggle. As he continued, within a few feet he noticed a swarm of ants cutting up the beautiful butterfly into pieces and carrying them into their ant hole. What happened he wondered?

This is what really happened. Nature took its course. The struggle that butterflies go through when coming out of their cocoons is what allows the body fluids to go to all their extremities and develop the strength they will need to fly, otherwise they will be too weak to fly away and become victims or the other predators of nature. Had not the man cut the cocoon and allowed the butter to struggle as required by nature, it would have been able to fly instead of become a feast for the ants. The moral of the story: Struggles is what makes us strong in life!

With that said, our bodies require exercise and stretching to become toned and strong. Those exercises promote proper circulation and strengthening of the heart. In today's modern era, we drive, sit, and are inactive too much to get the proper movement our body was designed to do. How many times do you drive half a block to the store or to visit a neighbor instead of walking? Even changing the channel on the television becomes bothersome. You need the darn remote!

We want everything made simple and easy. No wonder obesity and heart disease have gotten worse as exercise and simple tasks have been reduced to small physical efforts. Pushing buttons or programming tasks have dominated the present and perhaps the future. Therefore, we need to make time to exercise and strengthen our body, healthy mind-set, and heart. It should not even be an option, it should be a requirement.

TAKING RISKS

I recall seeing a poster at a doctor's office which had a beautiful boat at a dock. The poster had a message. It read, "It may look great on a dock but that is not its purpose". How true this is. Sometimes we feel that we need to live in a comfort would have not happened had nobody taken risks and have the courage to wander off their comfort zone. So it is when trying something new or different. As small or big it might seem at the time, a risk is required. I recall the time I decided to go to college about three hundred miles from home. It was my first the first time I was going to be away from my parents. I was going to a place where I was going to be where I knew nobody, not know what to expect, and be on my own to a large degree. I took the risk because I wanted to play college basketball. The opportunity I always wanted was placed at my feet but with strings attached. The strings came with risks. I had an experience I will always cherish and remember. I have no regrets. In fact, I am happy I made the decision I made. Not all risks guarantee success or positive outcomes. They all, however, provide a gain of courage. All failures only get you closer to success. Insanity is defined as doing the same thing over and over and over without success. Moral; learn from failures and try something different.

Without risks, America would not have been discovered by the natives that Leif Erickson or Columbus found on this continent. Neil Armstrong would have never stepped on the moon and opened the gates for space travel if the Wright brothers not risked their flight dreams. I can go on and on. I think you get the picture. How far you get in accomplishing your dreams boils down to how many risks you are willing to take. So, get off your comfort zone and take a risk and join me in your new venture and important dream and acquire a great healthy body and a healthy diet! My favorite poem designed for 'dream killers' or 'HATERS' as I call them was written by Mother Teresa, one of the most humble and giving individuals to walk this Earth. She also had the love, compassion, and courage paraphrase her poem.

DO IT ANYWAY!
People are illogical, unreasonable, and self-centered
Love them ANYWAY,
If you do good, you will be accused of doing it for selfish motives,
Do good ANYWAY,
When you succeed, envious individuals will hate you,
Succeed ANYWAY,
The good you do today, will be forgotten by tomorrow,
Do good ANYWAY,
Honesty and truthfulness will make you vulnerable,
Be honest and truthful ANYWAY,
The best individuals with the best ideas and dreams will be ridiculed,
Pursue your best ideas and dreams ANYWAY,
People usually pull for the underdog but follow the Top Dog,
Always fight for the underdogs ANYWAY
What you have spend most of your life building might be destroyed overnight
Build ANYWAY,
People may attack you for helping and standing up for those in need,
Help ANYWAY,
Give the world the best you can even if you get kicked in the process,
Give the world the best of yourself ANYWAY,
AT THE END, IT WAS BETWEEN YOU AND GOD ANYWAY!
(Paraphrased; Mother Teresa)

CHAPTER IV.

BECOMING THE BADASS
(TRUSTING AND BUILDING YOUR SELF-CONFIDENCE)

The first thing we usually look at to see how we look is our reflection, whether in the mirror or glass. Next time you want to see yourself, go to the mirror and really take a good look. That is also how others see the other you. Our appearance matters quite a bit. Ask a woman before she starts to put on her make-up, choose her clothes and shoes. A man is not as picky, but to a degree, also does his best to look presentable. One, therefore, can conclude that we as individuals care about how others also see us.

As a small child, I recall that even in school, our appearance mattered. Some of the kids were quick to label others by their appearance. Nicknames were used to criticize our looks. Most of them were negative; 'Fatso, 'Skinny, 'Elephant-eared', 'Darkie', etc., were born out of the first form of criticism. The result we refer to it as poor self-esteem. Unfortunately, it's only the beginning of the destruction of the inner emotional individual. Emotions can overcome and overpower an individual's daily performance and activities. Low self-esteem ridicule, depression, and loneliness are the top reasons why people visit psychiatrists and counselors.

I recall a story of a young boy who suffered from a bad case of rickets, a bow-legged deformity caused by lack of vitamin D in early childhood. His rickets was so severe he had to wear braces so he walk and also assist his legs to grow properly. While in school he was ridiculed and poked fun at. As he got older, he developed a bad inferior complex because of his deformity. He withdrew and allowed himself to have a defeated attitude. He, like all kids, had dreams of becoming a great football player. His favorite football player and idol in life was Jim Brown who was one of the best running backs of his era. He also had a small poster of his favorite player where he shared his bedroom with his siblings. Jim Brown was to become a legend and future Hall of Famer. One day, he found out that Jim Brown, of the Cleveland Browns, was going to be in Los Angeles to play the then Los Angeles Rams. The little boy, who lived in Los Angeles, made plans and asked his single parent mom if he could go. His mom told him that they could not afford the ticket for the game and to forget about making plans for attending the game. The kid begged and finally convinced his mom by promising her that he would only go and wait until after the game because all he wanted was to get a glimpse of Jim Brown. His plan was to wait until the game ended and he would sneak in and hide where the player's bus was parked and waited for Jim Brown to come out of visitors and get a real life glimpse of his idol. The big day came and the little boy walked almost cross town to the stadium where the game was to be played. He waited until the moment came. The game ended and the crowds found themselves out of the stadium. He ran into the parking area when the security guards were not watching. The kid hid under the bleachers until he saw the visiting football players starting to exit the dressing rooms and climb into the bus that would take them to the airport. Finally Jim Brown exited the dressing room and as he walked towards the bus, the young eight year old limped unto his path and pulled out his small poster of his idol and a pen. Brown was surprised but very cordial especially because of his physical deformity. The little boy extended his hand and asked if he could sign his poster. Brown shook his hand, took the poster and autographed it. Brown smiled and brushed his hand over his head and started to walk away when the little boy shouted at him, "One day I'm gonna break your records sir". Jim Brown was amused by the brave and alarming words of this young boy with braces on his legs.

Jim Brown turned around and smiled and replied, "Really, so what's your name so I can remember when you do?" The little boy answered, "Orthal, Orthal James ". Orthal James grew up and worked on his leg muscles by running and running. His determination and confidence changed his life. He was able to have his removed. As a freshman in high school he ran track and impressed his coaches. He tried out for football his sophomore year and made the varsity. He broke Jim Brown's high school rushing records. He earned a college scholarship to play football and track at the University of Southern California (USC) where he broke Jim Brown's college rushing records. He even out did Jim Brown collegiate records by winning the coveted HEISMAN TROPHY. He was drafted by the Buffalo Bills and broke Jim Brown's professional rushing records. Jim Brown made sure he attended the game when Orthal broke his record in a snowy game. After the game, it is said that Jim Brown went into the dressing room to personally congratulate Orthal James, or better known as O.J. Simpson!

Self acceptance at times can be a huge obstacle to overcome. You are who you are. The real you lay beneath what you see in the mirror. Only you can decide to change the outer you. Some individuals go to plastic surgeons, have dangerous medical procedures done to lose body fat, or have added body content to enhance key body parts. Most, however, take the smart, safer, and healthy way; exercise and healthy lifestyles. I have seen individuals lose over two hundred pounds just by exercising. How they feel about themselves afterwards is just amazing. Their self esteem soars, their energy level rises, and their emotional stress just about disappears but strengthens the once thin emotional coat. Ridicule, criticism, and self negative must be defeated. Only you can defeat and overcome your personal greatest fears, monsters, and negativities in your life.

On the other hand, vanity can be just as destructive. Vanity and bigotry are as one. Bigotry simply means feeling superior to others. Nobody likes the 'me, me, me' individuals whose first word out of their mouth is either 'I' o 'me'. In God's eyes, we are all equal and are part of His creation. Each one of us has the duty to accept ourselves for who we are.) However, we do have the **potential** (haven't done it yet) to become the best we can be! We were placed here to become winners not losers. Although our outer appearance seems to dominate on whether we accept ourselves or not, it is the inner-self that needs to overcome and dominate. In the most frankness way, we have to learn is to 'give a *sh__!*' how people think of us. But on the same level, accept others and treat others with utmost respect. Always use the Golden Rule; Not the one that refers to the evil one who says that "He who has the Gold makes the rules", but rather the one given to us by the Almighty, **"Treat others as one would like to be treated"**. Humbleness is one of the keys to happiness. Giving of yourself to others compliments humbleness and rewards your soul or inner self. They will provide a positive inner energy or force that will give you the confidence and desire to continue being the person you want to be and were meant to be.

Another key is how you carry yourself. Smile often and stop to smell the coffee or flowers ---- which ever turns you on. Take deep breaths and enjoy the life and healthy body you have been blessed with. Take time to listen to your inner sounds of the heart and your lungs at work. Enjoy the vivid colors that come to your mind as you close your eyes when you give them rest. And as you relax try to erase all the negativity that crossed your path during the day. Meditate or pray and count your blessings instead of sheep. Enjoy the 'greatest machine' that you are; a human body!

IMPORTANT TO KNOW

Cross Training and Exercise Circuit Training

Cross Training the style of fitness in which you will be using. It consists of utilizing different and various kinds of training exercises that will benefit for what is best of available and designed exercises. In other words, instead of only sticking to one type of exercise whether weights, running, stretching, power lifting, or others, Cross Training takes the best suited to target required to attain the muscle tone needed. Not one specific training program is used rather different exercises from various training programs are used to attain goal.

Exercise Circuit is a series of exercises in which is considered to be a group or numerous exercises in which the individual must do to compete a full circle and restart them again if required by the program. **In this program,** for example, an individual might start with a set of bench for 8 reps, bicep curls for 8 reps, push ups for 10 reps then finish with 12 triceps' extensions, etc. Once he/she finishes the cycle that is considered a circuit or round. Usually, it is recommended that there be 30 to ninety seconds between each exercise as the rest ratio. After your short rest, you can begin the second circuit or round till you're done with the number of circuits the workout calls for. You don't want to rest too long between each exercise because you need to continue before the muscle gets too relaxed. It is recommended no more than 2-3 minutes between circuits. This will allow your body to burn more fat metabolically and stimulate the muscles focused. The success will be determined by you commitment, focus, and carrying out the plan. The level of fitness for being in great shape for this program is completing 2-3 rounds, Elite or a fitness badass, is finishing the whole workout. Good luck

"EVERY MORNING IN AFRICA, A GAZELLE WAKES UP. IT KNOWS IT MUST OUTRUN THE FASTEST LION OR IT WILL BE KILLED. EVERY MORNING IN AFRICA, A LION WAKES UP. IT KNOWS IT MUST RUN FASTER THAN THE SLOWEST GAZELLE,OR IT WILL STARVE TO DEATH. IT DOESN'T MATTER WHETHER YOUR'RE A LION OR GAZELLE-WHEN THE SUN COMES UP YOU'D BETTER BE RUNNING."

-ROGER BANNISTER

HOW TO BE A FITNESS BADASS

THIS VI WEEK EXERCISE PROGRAM AND 30 DAY MEAL PLAN WAS DEVELOPED BY FORMER FITNESS WORLD CHAMPION AND FORMER FITNESS TRAINER AND ST. LOUIS CARDINALS STRENGTH STAFF MEMBER JACOB "HOLLYWOOD" HOWELL TO DEVELOP SPECIFIC STRENGTH AND BODY MECHANICS. THESE CROSS TRAINING EXERCISES WILL CONSTRUCT YOUR BODY TO BE AN ELITE ATHLETE THATS A LEAN, BADASS FITNESS MACHINE. YOU WILL BE GIVEN THE TOOLS AND BLUE PRINT TO TAKE YOUR FITNESS TO ANOTHER LEVEL USING THE ART OF FITNESS OF CROSS TRAINING & STRENGTH & CONDITIONING.

THE PHASES
THE THREE PHASES OF BEING A FITNESS BADASS CONSIST OF:

PHASE I: HYPERTROPHY/
MUSCLE ENDURANCE TWO WEEK OF 75% OF MAX

PHASE II: BASIC STRENGTH TWO WEEKS OF 85% OF MAX

PHASE III: STRENGTH AND POWER TWO WEEKS 90-95% OF MAX & A OVER LOAD PEROID

CROSS TRAIN: IMPLEMENTING WEIGHS WITH A COMBINATION OF DIFFERENT EXERCISES AND CONDITIONING OPTIONS SUCH HAS SPORTS PLAY,BIKING,JUMP ROPE AND COMBINING THESE EXERCISES WILL HELP YOU TRAIN LIKE A ATHLETE AND BECOME A TOTAL BADASS!

BODY CHECKS

NAME	WEEK I	WEEK VI	
HEGHT			
WEIGHT			
FAT%			
WAIST SIZE			

B E N C H	SQUAT	CLEAN	PUSH UP	VERT.	PULL UP	SIT UPS	1.5 MILE RUN	DATE

BODY WEIGHT	DATE	

How to become a fitness BADASS

the Vi week Workout

PHASE I WK I-II

HOW TO BE A FITNESS BADASS
CROSS –TRAINING FOR ELITE ATHLETES

CROSS-TRAINING	LOWER BODY	3-1 TEMPO	HYPERTROPHY/ ENDURANCE
MONDAY WK 1-2 75% OF MAX/ 3 SETS OF 6-12	SETS/REPS	*TEMPO EXAMPLE OF 3-1 IS 3 SEC DOWN OR NEGATIVE AND 1 SEC UP EXPLOSION	WEIGHT 75%
BACK SQUATS 75% MAX	3x12		
POWER CLEANS	3X6		
LEG EXTENSIONS	3X12	**CORE WORK**	**CONDITIONING**
DUMBBELL SQUAT JUMPS	3X12	TOE TOUCHES 4X20	4x200yds 4x50yds SPRINTS

CROSS-TRAINING	UPPER BODY	3-1 TEMPO	
TUESDAY WK 1-2	SETS/REPS	3 SEC DOWN NEGATIVE,1 SEC UP EXPLOSION	
BENCH PRESS	4X10		**CONDITIONING**
INCLINE PRESS	3X10	SIT UPS 4X20	4X200yds SPRINTS
SHOULDER-PRESS	3X10	**CORE WORK**	BIKE RIDE 5 MILES
PUSH-UPS	3X12	SIT UPS 4X20	OR
TRICEP DIPS	3X12	CRUNCHES 2X12	SPORT PLAY
PULL UPS	3X10		45 MIN- 1HR

PHASE I WK I

SPRINT WORK	CONDTIONING	3-1 TEMPO	HYPERTROPHY/ ENDURANCE
WED WK 1-2	SETS/REPS	3 SEC DOWN NEGATIVE,1 SEC UP EXPLOSION	
400	X1		
300	X1		
200	X2		
100	X2		**CONDITIONING**
5 MIN COOL DOWN STRETCH		**CORE WORK**	1.5- 2 MILE JOG
		PUSH UPS 4X12	
		CRUNCHES 4X20	

CROSS TRAINING	TOTAL BODY	3-1 TEMPO	HYPERTROPHY/ENDURANCE
THUR WK 1	SETS/REPS	3 SEC DOWN NEGATIVE,1 SEC UP EXPLOSION	WEIGHT 75-80%
LUNCHES	3X12		
BICEP CURLS	3X12		
PUSH UP	3X20	**CORE WORK**	**SPORT PLAY**
DB INCLINE BENCH	3X12	SIT UPS 4X20	45 MIN- 1HR
SHOULDER PRESS	3X12	PLANKS 3X30 SEC.	EXAMPLE:TENNIS
BACK ROW	3X12		

FRIDAY-SAT	SPORT PLAY	1 HR

"THE STRONGEST OAK OF THE FOREST IS NOT THE ONE THAT IS PROTECTED FROM THE STORM AND HIDDEN FROM THE SUN. IT'S THE ONE THAT STANDS IN THE OPEN WHERE IT IS COMPELLED TO STRUGGLE FOR IT'S EXISTENCE AGAINST THE WINDS AND RAINS AND SCORCHING SUN."

-NAPOLEON HILL

PHASE I WK II

CROSS TRAIN CIRCUIT	TOTAL BODY	TEMPO 2-1	HYPERTROPHY/ENDURANCE
MONDAY WK 1-2 75-% OF MAX	SETS/REPS	2 SEC DOWN NEGATIVE,1 SEC UP EXPLOSION	WEIGHT 75-80%
SQUATS 75% MAX	3X10-12		
SPLIT CLEAN	3X5		
BOX JUMPS	3X12	**CORE WORK**	**CONDITIONING**
INCLINE PRESS	4X12	PLANKS 3X30 SEC	BICYCLE RIDE 3 MILE
DIPS	4X-12	SIT UPS 3X20	SPORTS PLAY
PULL UPS	4X12	BICYCLES 3X30	45 MIN- 1HR

CONDITIONING	SPEED DAY		
TUESDAY WK 1-2	SETS/REPS		
DYNAMIC STRETCH	5MIN		
300 YDS	X2		
200 YDS	X3	**CORE WORK**	
100 YDS	X2	CRUNCHES 3X20	
		SIT UPS 3X12	
		TRUNK TWIST 3X20	

PHASE I WK II

CROSS TRAINING	UPPER BODY	2-1 TEMPO	HYPERTROPHY/ENDURANCE
WED WK 1-2 75-80%	SETS/REPS	2 SEC DOWN NEGATIVE,1 SEC UP EXPLOSION	WEIGHT 80% 1RM
BENCH PRESS	4X8	SUPER STATION	
INCLINE BENCH	3X8		
LAT PULL DOWNS	3X12		
PUSH UPS	3X12	**CORE WORK**	**CONDITIONING**
MACHINE CHEST PRESS	3X12	PLANKS 3X 1MIN	JUMP ROPE 15 MIN
DUMBBELL ROW	3X12	TRUNK TWIST 3X20	STEP MASTER 10 MIN
BICEP CURL	3X12	TOE TOUCHES 3X12	SPORTS PLAY 45 MIN
TRICEP DIPS	3X12	SIT UPS 3X20	EX: BASKETBALL

CROSS TRAIN	LOWER BODY	2-1 TEMPO	HYPERTROPHY/ENDURANCE
THUR WK 1-2	SETS/REPS	2 SEC DOWN NEGATIVE,1 SEC UP EXPLOSION	WEIGHT 75-80%
SQUAT 80% SUPER SET WITH WALKING LUNGE	4X8 ON SQUAT 3X12 ON LUNGES		
FRONT SQUAT	3X12 (LIGHT)	**CORE WORK**	**CONDITIONING**
BOX STEP UPS		SIT UPS 3X12	
WALKING LUNGE		TRUNK TWIST 3X12	JUMP ROPE 15 MIN
BOX JUMPS	3X12	PLANKS 5X.30 SECONDS	STATIONARY BIKE 25 MIN

FRIDAY-SAT	RECOVER	REST

**HOW TO BE A FITNESS BADASS
CROSS –TRAINING FOR ELITE ATHLETES**

PHASE II WK III-IV

CROSS TRAINING	LOWER BODY	2-1 TEMPO	BASIC STRENGTH
MONDAY WK 3-4 85% OF MAX	SETS/REPS	2 SEC DOWN NEGATIVE,1 SEC UP EXPLOSION	WEIGHT 85-90%
SQUATS	4X6		
POWER CLEANS	4X6	**CORE WORK**	**CONDITIONING**
BOX STEP UPS	3X20	PLANKS 4X.30 SECONDS	JUMP ROPE 10- MIN
HAMSTRING CURLS (MACHINE)	3X20	CRUNCHES 3X30	STATIONARY BIKE 45 MIN
KETTLE BELL SQUAT JUMPS	3X20	TOE TOUCHES 3X30	UP HILL SPRINTS 5X35 YDS

		TEMPO 2-1	
TUESDAY WK 3 BADASS CONDITIONING 75-80% FULL SPEED	SPEED DAY TRACK DAY	2 SEC DOWN NEGATIVE,1 SEC UP EXPLOSION	
DYNAMIC STRETCH	5MIN		
400 M	X1		
200 M	X3	**CORE WORK**	**CONDITIONING**
100 M	X3	CRUNCHES 3X20	BIKE RIDE 45 MIN
50 M	X3	SIT UPS 3X20	
COOL DOWN STRETCH	5 MIN	TOE TOUCHES 3X20	

"I'VE MISSED MORE THAN 9,000 SHOTS IN MY CAREER AND HAVE LOST MORE THAN 300 GAMES. I'VE BEEN TRUSTED TO TAKE THE GAME WINNING SHOT 26 TIMES AND HAVE FAILED OVER AND OVER AGAIN. AND THATS WHY I SUCCEED."

-MICHAEL JORDAN

PHASE II WK IV

CROSS TRAINING	UPPER BODY	TEMPO 2-1	HYPERTROPHY/ENDURANCE
WED WK 3-4	SETS/REPS	2 SEC DOWN NEGATIVE,1 SEC UP EXPLOSION	
INCLINE BENCH SUPER SET WITH PUSH UPS	4X12 ON BENCH 4X20 ON PUSH UPS		
PULL-UPS	4X12		
DIPS	4X12		
BI CURL (BAR)	4X8	**CORE WORK**	**CONDITIONING**
SHOULDER PRESS (BAR)	3X8	BICYLE KICKS 4X20	BOX JUMPS 5X20
DB FLYS	3X12	SIT UPS 4X20	JUMP ROPE 5 MIN
DB ROWS	3X12	TOE TOUCHES 4X20	STATIONARY BIKE 30 MIN

CROSS TRAINING	LOWER BODY	2-1 TEMPO	HYPERTROPHY/ENDURANCE
THUR WK 4	SETS/REPS	2 SEC DOWN NEGATIVE,1 SEC UP EXPLOSION	WEIGHT 90%
SQUAT 90% SUPER SET WITH DEAD LIFT	4X5 ON (HEAVY) SQUAT 4X12 ON DEAD LIFT (LIGHT)	**CORE WORK**	**CONDITIONING**
FRONT SQUAT	3X5	CRUNCHES 4X20	STATION BIKE 25 MIN
MACHINE HAMSTRING CURLS	3X20	TRUNK TWIST 4X20	UP HILL SPRINTS 5X30 YDS
WALKING LUNGE	3X20 STEPS	TOE TOUCH 4X20	

PHASE II WK IV-V

CROSS TRAINING	UPPER BODY	TEMPO 2-1	HYPERTROPHY/ENDURANCE
MONDAY WK 3-4	SETS/REPS	2 SEC DOWN NEGATIVE,1 SEC UP EXPLOSION	
DB BENCH	4X12		
DB SHOULDER PRESS	4X12		
DIPS SUPER SET WITH PUSH UPS	3X15 ON DIPS 3X15 ON PUSH UPS		
BI CURL (BAR)	4X12	**CORE WORK**	**CONDITIONING**
BOX SQUATS	3X12	TOE TOUCHES 4X25	STATIONARY BIKE 30 MIN
WALKING LUNGE	3X12	PLANKS 4X.30 SECONDS	STEP MASTER 10 MIN
HAMSTRING CURLS	3X12	CRUNCHES 4X25	

FRIDAY-SAT	SPORTS PLAY	1- HOUR

REST & RECOVER

THE NEXT FEW DAYS IN THIS **PHASE.** WORKOUT IN WEEK 5,WHICH IS UP COMING UP NEXT WEEK KEEP UP THE GREAT AMAZING WORK. THIS IS THE POINT MOST PEOPLE QUIT, BUT NOT YOU!!!!!!

"HOW DOES ONE BECOME A BUTTERFLY? YOU MUST WANT TO FLY SO MUCH THAT YOU ARE WILLING TO GIVE UP BEING A CATERPILLAR."

-TRINA PAULUS

PHASE II WK VI

CROSS TRAINING	LOWER BODY	2-1 TEMPO	STRENGTH/POWER
MONDAY WK 5 90-95% OF MAX/ 3X3-5	SETS/REPS	2 SEC DOWN NEGATIVE,1 SEC UP EXPLOSION	WEIGHT 90-95%
SQUATS	5X5 (HEAVY)		
MACHINE LEG PRESS	5X5 (HEAVY)		
BOX STEP UPS	3X15	**CORE WORK**	**CONDITIONING**
MACHINE LEG EXTENTION	3X15	TRUNK TWIST 4X25	STATIONARY BIKE 20 MIN
WALKING LUNGE	3X20 STEPS	BICYCLE KICKS 4X25	STEP MASTER 20 MIN
BOX JUMPS	2X15	SIT UPS 4X25	JUMP ROPE 5 MIN

CROSS TRAINING	UPPER BODY	2-1 TEMPO	STRENGTH/POWER
TUES WK 5	SETS/REPS	2 SEC DOWN NEGATIVE,1 SEC UP EXPLOSION	WEIGHT 90-95%
BENCH 90-95% -S	5X3-5		
INCLINE BENCH	4X12		
BI CURL	4X8	**CORE WORK**	**CONDITIONING**
CABLE LAT PULL DOWN	3X12	PLANKS 5X.30 SEC	SPRINTS
DB SHOULDER PRESS	3X12	TOE TOUCHES 3X25	10X100 YDS REST 45 SEC BETWEEN SPRINTS
PULL UPS	4X12	SIT UPS 3X25	400 METER COOL DOWN JOG

PHASE II WK VI heavy load

CROSS TRAINING	LOWER BODY	3-1 TEMPO	STRENGTH/POWER
WED WK 5 90-95% OF MAX/ 3X3-5	SETS/REPS	3 SEC DOWN NEGATIVE,1 SEC UP EXPLOSION	WEIGHT 90-95%
SQUATS	5x3 (HEAVY)		
MACHINE LEG CURLS	5X8 (HEAVY)		
LUNGE	3X12 STEPS	CORE WORK	CONDITIONING
POWER CLEANS	5X5	SIT UPS 3X25	UP HILL SPRINTS 5X35 YDS
MACHINE LEG PRESS	3X5 (HEAVY)	CRUNCHES 3X25	TRAIL RUN/JOG 35 MIN
MACHINE HAMSTRING CURLS	3X12	TRUNK TWIST 3X25	

CROSS TRAINING	UPPER BODY	3-1 TEMPO	STRENGTH/POWER
THUR WK 5		3 SEC DOWN NEGATIVE,1 SEC UP EXPLOSION	WEIGHT 90-95%
BENCH 90-95% -S	5X5 (HEAVY)		
INCLINE BENCH	3X5 (HEAVY)		
BI CURL	3X8	**CORE WORK**	**CONDITIONING**
DB PEC PRESS	3X6 (HEAVY)	TRUNK TWIST 5X30	BIKE RIDE 5 MILES
SHOULDER PRESS	3X6 (HEAVY)	SIT UPS 3X30	
LAT PULL DOWN	3X12	CRUNCHES 3X30	

FRIDAY-SAT	*RECOVER*	*REST*

" PAIN IS TEMPORARY. IT MAY LAST A MINUTE, OR AN HOUR,OR A DAY, OR A YEAR, BUT EVENTUALLY IT WILL SUBSIDE AND SOMETHING ELSE WILL TAKE ITS PLACE. IF I QUIT, HOWEVER, IT WILL LAST FOREVER."

-LANCE ARMSTRONG

PHASE II
FITNESS BADASS
MAX TEST

MAX TEST	PHASE 2 RESULTS
BENCH	
SQUAT	
PUSH UP REPS	
PULL UPS REPS	
1.5 MILE TIME	
BODY WEIGHT	

PHASE III START NEW CYCLE

HOW TO BE A FITNESS BADASS
CROSS –TRAINING FOR ELITE ATHLETES

PHASE III WK I-II

CROSS TRAINING	LOWER BODY	2-1 TEMPO	STRENGTH/POWER
MONDAY WK 1-2 90-95% OF MAX/ 3X3-5	SETS/REPS	2 SEC DOWN NEGATIVE,1 SEC UP EXPLOSION	
SQUATS	5X3 (HEAVY)		
BAR STEP UPS	4X12		
WALKING LUNGE	3X12	**CORE WORK**	**CONDITIONING**
HAMSTRING CURLS	4X20	BICYCLE KICKS 4X25	STATIONARY BIKE 45-50 MIN
FRONT SQUAT	3X20 (LIGHT)	TOE TOUCHES 4X25	
DB CLEAN	3X5-6	PLANKS 4X 1 MIN	

		3-1 TEMPO	
TUESDAY WK 1	UPPER BODY SETS/REPS	3 SEC DOWN NEGATIVE,1 SEC UP EXPLOSION	
DB BENCH	5X5 (HEAVY)		
INCLINE BENCH	5X5 (HEAVY)	**CORE WORK**	**CONDITIONING**
BICEP MACHINE	4X20	TRUNK TWIST 3X20	STEP MASTER 35 MIN
TRICEP PULL DOWN	4X20	PLANKS 4X 1MIN	JUMP ROPE 5 MIN
DB BACK ROW	4X12	SIT UPS 3X25	
SHOULDER PRESS	3X5-6 (HEAVY)	BICYCLE KICKS 3X25	

PHASE III WK I

CROSS TRAINING	UPPER BODY	2-1 TEMPO	STRENGTH/POWER
WED WK 1 90-95% 3X 5-3	SETS/REPS	2 SEC DOWN NEGATIVE,1 SEC UP EXPLOSION	
BENCH 90-95%	SUPER SET WITH INCLINE 5X5 (HEAVY)		
LAT PULL DOWN	5X15		
DB BICEPT CURL	5X15	**CORE WORK**	**CONDITIONING**
SHOULDER PRESS /PUSH UP	SUPER SET WITH PUSH UPS 5X10	TOE TOUCHES 5X30	SPRINTS 5X50 YDS
DIPS & BI CURL	SUPER SET 3X12	TRUNK TWIST 3X30	SPRINTS 5X30 YDS
DB BACK ROW	3X12		

LOWER BODY		3-1 TEMPO	
THUR WK 1	SETS/REPS	3 SEC DOWN NEGATIVE,1 SEC UP EXPLOSION	
BOX SQAUT	5X3-5 (HEAVY)	**CORE WORK**	**CONDITIONING**
HAM STRING CURL	3X20	BICYCLE KICKS 3X30	UP HILL SPRINT 5X35 YDS
LEG EXTENSION MACHINE	3X20	PLANKS 5X .30 SEC	JOG 20 MIN
WALKING LUNGE	5X10 STEPS	CRUNCHES 5X30	

FRIDAY-SAT	**SPORTS PLAY**	**1 HOUR**

"NINETY-NINE PERCENT OF THE FAILURES COME FROM PEOPLE WHO HAVE THE HABIT OF MAKING EXCUSES."

-GEORGE WASHINGTON CARVER

PHASE III WK II

CROSS TRAINING	LOWER BODY	2-1 TEMPO	SPEED PHASE
MONDAY WK 2 75-80% 3X 10-12	SETS/REPS	2 SEC DOWN NEGATIVE,1 SEC UP EXPLOSION	
SQUATS 75-80%	3X12		
BOX JUMPS	3X12		
DB LUNGE	3X25	**CORE WORK**	**CONDITIONING**
POWER CLEAN	3X6	BYCYCLE KICKS 3X30	STATIONARY BIKE 20 MIN
HAMSTRING CURL	3X25	PLANKS 5X 1MIN	BOX JUMPS 5X12
		SIT UPS 3X30	JUMP ROPE 5 MIN

TUES WK 2	UPPER BODY	3-1 TEMPO	
WK 2 75-80% 5-3X	SETS/REPS	3 SEC DOWN NEGATIVE,1 SEC UP EXPLOSION	
BENCH PRESS	3X12		
BI CURL	5X12		
INCLINE	3X25	**CORE WORK**	**CONDITIONING**
DIPS	5X12	CRUNCHES 5X30	
DB SHOULDER PRESS	3X12	TOE TOUCHES 5X30	SPORTS PLAY 45 MIN

PHASE III WK II-III

WED WK 2	UPPER BODY	2-1 TEMPO	STRENGTH/POWER
		2 SEC DOWN NEGATIVE,1 SEC UP EXPLOSION	
BENCH 80-85 % -S			
INCLINE BENCH	X12		
BI CURL		**CORE WORK**	**CONDITIONING**
DB BALL INCLINE			
SHOULDER PRESS			
DIPS			

CONDITIONING	SPEED DAY		
THUR WK 1-2	SETS/REPS		
DYNAMIC STRETCH	5MIN		
300 YDS	X3		
200 YDS	X3	**CORE WORK**	
100 YDS	X2	CRUNCHES 3X20	
		SIT UPS 3X12	
		TRUNK TWIST 3X20	

"THERE IS NO LIMIT TO WHAT YOU CAN IMAGINE. AND WITH COMMITMENT AND EFFORT, WHAT YOU CAN IMAGINE, YOU CAN BECOME. PUT YOUR MIND TO WORK FOR YOU. BELIEVE THAT YOU CAN DO IT. THE WORLD WILL TELL YOU THAT YOU CAN'T. YET IN YOUR BELIEFS YOU'LL FIND THE STRENGTH, YOU'LL FIND THE ABILITY TO DO IT ANYWAY."

-RALPH MARSTON

PHASE III WK III

CROSS TRAINING	LOWER BODY	3-1 TEMPO	STRENGTH/POWER
MONDAY WK 3 90-95% OF MAX/ 3X3-5		3 SEC DOWN NEGATIVE,1 SEC UP EXPLOSION	
BOX SQUATS			
SQUAT JUMPS			
WALKING LUNGE		**CORE WORK**	**CONDITIONING**
POWER CLEAN		CRUNCHES 5X30	
DEAD LIFT		SIT UPS 5X30	
		CRUNCHES 3X30	

TUES WK 3	UPPER BODY	2-1 TEMPO	STRENGTH/POWER
FLOOR PRESS 90-95% 3X5		3 SEC DOWN NEGATIVE,1 SEC UP EXPLOSION	
INCLINE BENCH			
BI CURL			
BENCH PRESS		**CORE WORK**	**CONDITIONING**
BALL INCLINE			
DIPS/PUSH UPS			
BACK WORK			

PHASE III WK III

CROSS TRAINING	UPPER BODY	2-1 TEMPO	STRENGTH/POWER
WED WK 3 90-95% 3X5	SETS X3	2 SEC DOWN NEGATIVE,1 SEC UP EXPLOSION	
BENCH 90-95 % -S			
INCLINE BENCH			
BI CURL		**CORE WORK**	**CONDTIONING**
DB BALL INCLINE			TRAIL RUN
SHOULDER PRESS			
CORE WORK			

THUR WK 3	LOWER BODY	3-1 TEMPO	STRENGTH/PO WER
SQUAT 90-95% 3X5-3		3 SEC DOWN NEGATIVE,1 SEC UP EXPLOSION	
LEG EXTENSIONS			
DEAD LIFT			
WALKING LUNGE		**CORE WORK**	**CONDTIONING**
DB HACK SQUAT			UP HILL SPRINTS 5X35 YDS
POWER CLEAN			JOG 20 MIN
BOX SQUATS			

FRIDAY-SAT	RECOVER	REST

"STRENGTH DOES NOT COME FROM WINNING. YOUR STRUGGLES DEVELOP YOUR STRENGTHS. WHEN YOU GO THROUGH HARDSHIPS AND DECIDE NOT TO SURRENDER, THAT IS STRENGTH."

-ARNOLD SCHWARZENEGGER

"FIGHT ONE MORE ROUND. WHEN YOUR ARMS ARE SO TIRED THAT YOU CAN HARDLY LIFT YOUR HANDS TO COME ON GUARD, FIGHT ONE MORE ROUND WHEN YOUR NOSE IS BLEEDING AND YOUR EYES ARE BLACK AND YOU ARE SO TIRED THAT YOU WISH YOUR OPPONENTS WOULD CRACK YOU ON THE JAW AND PUT YOU TO SLEEP, FIGHT ONE MORE ROUND - REMEMBERING THAT THE MAN WHO ALWAYS FIGHTS ONE MORE ROUND IS NEVER WHIPPED."

-JAMES CORBETT

PHASE III FINAL

FITNESS BADASS MAX TEST

MAX TEST	PHASE III RESULTS
BENCH	
SQUAT	
PUSH UP REPS	
PULL UPS REPS	
1.5 MILE TIME	
BODY WEIGHT	

THE 30 DAY HOW TO BE A FITNESS BADASS SAMPLE MEAL PLAN

"ITS A SHAME FOR A MAN TO GROW OLD WITHOUT SEEING THE BEAUTY AND STRENGTH OF WHICH HIS BODY IS CAPABLE."

SOCRATES

HOW TO BE A FITNESS BADASS FITNESS

*PROTEIN/CARBOHYDRATE POST- WORKOUT CALCULATOR

DAILY CALORIE INTAKE %
FOR A FITNESS BADASS

PROTEIN

ATHLETES WEIGHT (KG)
X .25g PROTEIN

10-15%
PROTEIN

=

RECOMMENDED PROTEIN
INTAKE POST-WORKOUT

20-35%
GOOD
FATS

CARBOHYDRATE

ATHLETES WEIGHT (KG)
X 1.0g CARBOHYDRATE

45-65%
CARBS

=

RECOMMENDED CARB INTAKE
POST-WORKOUT

* 1. SOURCE INFORMATION FOR PROTEIN/CARB CALCULATOR
GATORADE SPORTS SCIENCE INSTITUTE 2013
2. CALORIE INTAKE% NSCA 2012

HOW TO BE A FITNESS BADASS FITNESS NUTRITION TIPS

	%	EXAMPLES
PROTEINS	**45-65%**	LEAN MEATS: LEAN STEAK,FISH,CHICKEN,NUTSAND SOY BEANS. TRY EATING RED MEATS TO A MINIMUM.
CARBS	**10-15%**	EAT GOOD CARBS: WHEAT,GRAINS,FRUITS AND VEGETABLES. EXAMPLES: SALADS,GREEN PEPPER,GRAPES,APPLES AND MELONS
FATS	**20-35%**	EAT FATS??? WHAT, YOU MIGHT BE SAYING??? WELL GOOD FATS WILL DO YOUR BODY GOOD: OMEGA 3 FATS,FISH OIL,AVOCADOS, GRAPE SEED OIL AND OLIVE OIL. ALL THESE PROVIDE A EXCELLENT SOURCE OF GOOD FATS AND HELP THE BODYS HEART AND TISSUES, WHEN USED. AVOID SATURATED FAT COOKED FOODS FOUND IN BURGERS,FRIES AND FRY CHICKEN ETC.

HOW TO BE A FITNESS BADASS FITNESS NUTRITION TIPS

	PRE	POST
SPORTS NUTRITION TIP	EAT A LOW FAT HIGH PROTEIN MEAL 3-4 HOURS BEFORE EXERCISE WORKOUT TO FUEL YOUR BODY AND YOUR MUSCLES. ALSO TRY TO EAT 3 HEALTHY MEALS A DAY AND 2-3 SMALL HEALTHY SNACK BETWEEN YOUR MEALS TO PREVENT TISSUE BREAKDOWN AND TO HELP YOUR BODYS FAT METABOLISM.	TO HELP YOU RECOVER FROM THE WORKOUT, EAT NO LATER THEN 2-3 HOURS POST WORKOUT TO PREVENT MUSCLE BREAK DOWN. TRY A LOW FAT, HIGH PRTEIN MEAL WITH GOOD CARDS INCLUDED.
H20 (WATER) IS VERY IMPORTANT AND VITAL. THE AVG HUMAN BODY IS MADE OF 60-70% WATER. TRY TO DRINK AT LEAST 8 GLASSES OF WATER A DAY. ACTIVE ATHLETES SHOULD STAY AROUND 2 LITERS.	(1) ONE PINT OF WATER AT LEAST 2 HOURS BEFORE YOUR WORKOUT.	(1) ONE PINT OF WATER FOR EVERY POUND LOSS DURING THE END OF YOUR WORKOUT. THIS WILL HELP AVOIDS DEHYDRATION AND REPLENISH YOUR BODY.

*ALWAYS AVOID HIGH SUGAR AND HIGH CAFFEINE DRINKS AND DRINK PLENTY OF WATER THROUGH OUT THE DAY.

"NOTHING CAN STOP THE MAN WITH THE RIGHT MENTAL ATTITUDE FROM ACHIEVING HIS GOAL; NOTHING ON EARTH CAN HELP THE MAN WITH THE WRONG MENTAL ATTITUDE."

-THOMAS JEFFERSON

FITNESS BADASS SAMPLE 30 DAY MEAL PLAN

MEAL #1	SNACK	MEAL #2	SNACK	MEAL # 3
DAY 1 2 SCRAMBLED OR BOILED EGGS 1/2 GRAPE FRUIT	1 CUP GREEK YOGURT WITH 1/4 CUP OF MIXED BERRIES	6-8 OZ BAKED FISH & 1/2 CUP ROASTED RED POTATOES	1 APPLE , 1 OZ LOW FAT CHEESE	6-8 OZ GRILLED CHICKEN BREAST,1/2 CUP OF STEAMED VEGGIES
DAY 2 1 CUP OATMEAL WITH MIXED FRUIT,2 BOILED EGG	1/2 CUP COTTAGE CHEESE WITH CINNAMON OR FRUIT	1/2 TURKEY SANDWICH ,1 CUP LOW FAT SOUP	CELERY STICKS WITH 2 TBSP OF NATURAL PEANUT BUTTER	8 OZ GRILLED OR BROILED SALMON 1/2 SWEET POTATO
DAY 3 1 CUP OF GREEK YOGURT,1 CUP OF HIGH FIBER CEREAL	1/4 CUP OF MIXED NUTS OR LOW SUGAR TRAIL MIX	TURKEY MEAT BALLS SERVED OVER 1 CUP OF SPAGHETTI SQUASH WITH LIGHT SAUCE	1 RICE CAKE WITH 1 TBSP PEANUT BUTTER OR ALMOND BUTTER	8 OZ BAKED TILAPIA, 1 CUP STEAMED MIXED GREENS
DAY 4 EGG WHITE OMELET WITH 1 OZ LOW FAT OR FAT FREE CHEESE,1 SLICE WHEAT TOAST	1/4 CUP OF RAW MIXED NUTS	8 OZ CHICKEN CAESAR SALAD WITH FAT FREE DRESSING	1 CUP GREEK YOGURT WITH 1/4 CUP OF MIXED BERRIES	8 OZ BBQ CHICKEN BREAST, 1 CUP STEAMED BROCCOLI
DAY 5 1 CUP OF HIGH-FIBER CEREAL, 1/2 CUP OF FRUIT	1 CUP OF BAKED CINNAMON SLICES	6 0Z CANNED TUNA WITH 1 TBSP OF LIGHT MAYO, 1 SLICE OF WHEAT TOAST	2 SLICES OF LEAN DELI TURKEY BREAST	1/2 TURKEY BLT SANDWICH ON WHEAT, 1/2 CUP OF VEGGIE SOUP(LOW SODIUM)
DAY 6 2 POACHED EGGS,1/2 CUP OF OATMEAL WITH MIXED FRIUT	CARROT SLICES WITH 2 TBSP HUMMUS	1/4 SMOKED CHICKEN,1 CUP OF STEAMED GREENS	6-8 OZ GRILLED PORK CHOP WITH 1 CUP OF STEAMED OR GRILLED VEGGIES	GRILLED SHRIMP SALAD WITH FAT FREE DRESSING,1/2 OF COB OF STEAM CORN
DAY 7 LEAN STEAK EGG WHITE OMELET WITH LOW FAT CHEESE	1 RICE CAKE WITH 1 TBSP PEANUT BUTTER OR ALMOND BUTTER	6 OZ LEAN STEAK, 1/2 SWEET POTATOE	1 CUP OF LEAN BEEF CHILE	8 OZ SMOKED SALMON WITH 1/2 CUP STEAMED MIXED GREENS

MEAL #1	SNACK	MEAL #2	SNACK	MEAL # 3
DAY 8 2 POACHED EGGS WITH 1 SLICE OF CANADIAN BACON	1 SCOOP OF ISO-PROTEIN WITH 1/2 CUP OF FRUIT	8 OZ BAKED CODE,GRILLED VEGGIES OR MIXED GREENS	2 SLICE OF DELI TURKEY BREAST,1/2 CUP OF FRUIT	HERB GRILLED SHRIMP WITH ROASTED ASPARAGUS
DAY 9 1/2 CUP OF GREEK YOGURT WITH 1/4 CUP OF MIXED FRIUT AND 2 BOILED EGGS	1/2 CUP OF GREEK YOGURT AND 1/4 CUP OF FRUIT	6 OZ GRILLED LEAN PORK CHOP,1/2 COB OF GRILLED CORN	1 3-4 OZ CAN OF TUNA	CHICKEN FAJITA WRAP WITH GRILLED GREEN PEPPER ONION
DAY 10 1/2 CUP OF OATMEAL WITH 1/4 CUP OF APPLE SLICES AND 2 BOILED EGG	1/2 CUP OF MIXED FRIUT,1/4 CUP OF LOW FAT COTTAGE CHEESE	6 OZ TUNA CAN,1 CUP OF MIXED GREENS	1 HARD BOILED EGG AND 1 SLICE OF TURKEY JERKY	6 OZ SIRLOIN STEAK,1/2 BAKED SWEET POTATO OR SIDE OF 1 CUP OF BROWN RICE
DAY 11 2 SCRAMBLED EGGS WITH 2 SLICES OF TURKEY BACON	2 HARD BOILED EGGS	1 TURKEY SWISS SANDWICH ON WHEAT	1 SLICE OF WHEAT TOAST WITH 1 TBSB OF PEANUT BUTTER	6 OZ GRILLED CHICKEN BREAST,1 CUP OF STEAMED GREENS
DAY 12 EGG WHITE OMELET LOW FAT CHEESE	1 HARD BOILED EGG,1/2 APPLE SLICED WITH PEANUT BUTTER	8 OZ BAKED WHITE FISH WITH 1 CUP OF STEAMED GREENS	1/2 CUP OF GREEK YOGURT WITH 1/4 CUP OF MIXED FRIUT	8 OZ BAKED FISH,1 CUP OF STEAMED VEGGIES
DAY 13 1 CUP OF FIBER CEREAL 1 SCOOP OF ISO-PROTEIN WITH 1/2 CUP OF FRUIT	2 SLICES OF DELI TURKEY BREAST	8 OZ SLOW COOKED POT ROAST LEAN MEAT WITH 1/4 CUP OF ROASTED POTATOES	1 APPLE 2 SLICES OF TURKEY JERKY	6 OZ GRILLED LEAN PORK CHOP,1/2 COB OF GRILLED CORN
DAY 14 1/2 CUP OATMEAL WITH MIXED FRUIT,2 BOILED EGG	CHICKEN FAJITA WRAP WITH GRILLED GREEN PEPPER ONION	1/4 BAKE CHICKEN WITH SM SIDE SALAD	2 HARD BOILED EGGS	8-10 OZ STIR FRY MIXED WITH CHICKEN OR SHRIMP

MEAL #1	SNACK	MEAL #2	SNACK	MEAL # 3
DAY 15 2 SCRAMBLED EGGS WITH 1 ONCE OF LEAN HAM	1/2 CUP OF YOGURT	8 OZ GRILLED CHICKEN SERVED OVER 1 CUP OF GRILLED SQUASH	1/4 CUP OF RAW MIXED NUTS,LOW SODIUM	6 OZ GRILLED TUNA STEAK WITH FRESH GREEN SALAD
DAY 16 1 CUP OF OATMEAL WITH 1/2 CUP OF APPLE SLICES AND 1 BOILED EGG	6 SMALL CELERY STICKS WITH LOW FAT PEANUT BUTTER	TACO SALAD 8 OZ OF LEAN GROUND MEAT WITH 2 TBSB OF SOUR CREAM AND LOW FAT 1 OZ CHEESE	1/2 GRAPEFRUIT WITH 1 TURKEY JERKEY	6 COCONUT SHRIMP WITH 1/2 BAKED SWEET POTATO
DAY 17 2 POACHED EGGS 1/2 BOWL OF OATMEAL	1 RICE CAKE WITH 2 TBSP OF LOW FAT PEANUT BUTTER	1 BOWL ROASTED CHICKEN TOMATO SOUP	1 CUP OF FRUIT WITH 1/4 CUP OF COTTAGE CHEESE	8 OZ OF LEAN TURKEY LOAF,1 CUP OF STEAMED MIXED GREENS
DAY 18 1/2 BRAN MUFFIN AND 2 BOILED EGGS	1/2 CUP OATMEAL WITH MIXED FRUIT,1 BOILED EGG	8 OZ GRILLED SALMON WITH 1/4 OF AVOCADO	CELERY STICKS WITH 2 TBSP OF NATURAL PEANUT BUTTER	1 BOWL OF CHICKEN TOMATO SOUP
DAY 19 1/2 CUP OATMEAL WITH MIXED FRUIT,1 BOILED EGG	2 BOILED EGGS AND 1/2 A GRAPEFRUIT	1 CUP OF CHICKEN VEGETABLE SOUP, 1/4 BAKED CHICKEN	2 HARD BOILED EGGS,1/2 CUP OF FRUIT	1/4 BAKE CHICKEN WITH SM SIDE SALAD or 1 CUP RICE
DAY 20 1 CUP OF GREEK YOGURT AND 1/2 CUP OF FRIUT AND 2 BOILED EGGS	1 APPLE 2 SLICES OF TURKEY JERKEY	8 OZ PAN GRILLED FISH WITH 1 CUP OF STEAMED VEGGIES OR RICE	1 RICE CAKE WITH 2 TBSP OF LOW FAT PEANUT BUTTER	6 OZ GRILLED LEAN PORK CHOP,1/2 COB OF GRILLED CORN
DAY 21 2 POACHED EGGS WITH 1 SLICE OF CANADIAN BACON	1/2 CUP OF MIXED BERRIES AND 1/2 A CUP OF FAT FREE YOGURT	1 BOWL ROASTED CHICKEN TOMATO SOUP	1/2 CUP OATMEAL WITH MIXED FRUIT,1 BOILED EGG	8 OZ OVEN ROASTED CHICKEN WITH 1 CUP OF STEAMED GREENS

MEAL #1	SNACK	MEAL #2	SNACK	MEAL # 3
DAY 22 1/2 CUP OATMEAL WITH MIXED FRUIT,1 BOILED EGG	1 RICE CAKE WITH 2 TBSP OF LOW FAT PEANUT BUTTER	8 OZ BAKED COD FISH WITH 1 CUP OF STEAMED VEGGIES	1/2 CUP OF GREEK YOGURT AND 1/4 CUP OF FRIUT	8 OZ OVEN ROASTED CHICKEN WITH1 CUP OF STEAMED GREENS
DAY 23 1 CUP OF FIBER CEREAL 1 SCOOP OF ISO-PROTEIN WITH 1/2 CUP OF FRUIT	1/2 AVOCADO WITH 1 TURKEY JERKEY	8 OZ SLOW COOKED POT ROAST LEAN MEAT WITH 1/4 CUP OF ROASTED POTATOES	1/2 GRAPFRUIT 1 TURKEY JERKEY	6 OZ BAKED WHITE FISH WITH 1 CUP OF STEAMED GREENS
DAY 24 2 SCRAMBLED EGGS WITH 2 SLICES OF TURKEY BACON	2 SLICES OF DELI TURKEY BREAST	1 BOWL ROASTED CHICKEN TOMATO SOUP	1/2 CUP OATMEAL WITH MIXED FRUIT,1 BOILED EGG	BAKED TURKEY LEG WITH A SIDE OF STEAMED GREENS
DAY 25 1 OF CUP OATMEAL WITH 1/2 CUP OF MIXED FRUIT 2 BOILED EGG	2 HARD BOILED EGGS	6 OZ GRILLED LEAN PORK CHOP,1/2 COB OF GRILLED CORN	1 APPLE 2 SLICES OF TURKEY JERKEY	CHICKEN FAJITA WRAP WITH GRILLED GREEN PEPPER ONION
DAY 26 1 BOWL OF OATMEAL WITH 1/2 CUP OF BERRIES	1/2 CUP OF GREEK YOGURT AND 1/4 CUP OF FRIUT	8-10 OZ STIR FRY MIXED WITH CHICKEN OR SHRIMP	2 HARD BOILED EGGS	1 BOWL ROASTED CHICKEN TOMATO SOUP
DAY 27 EGG WHITE OMELET	1 APPLE 2 SLICES OF TURKEY JERKEY	8 OZ GRILLED SALMON WITH 1/4 OF AVOCADO WITH 1/2 CUP OF BROWN RICE	6 SMALL CELERY STICKS WITH LOW FAT PEANUT BUTTER	8 OZ PAN GRILLED FISH WITH 1/2 STEAMED VEGGIES
DAY 28 1 CUP OF GREEK YOGURT AND 1/2 CUP OF FRIUT AND 2 BOILED EGGS	1 SCOOP OF ISO-PROTEIN WITH 1/2 CUP OF FRUIT. Shake with fat-free milk and ½ cup of fruit	8 OZ PAN GRILLED FISH WITH 1 CUP OF STEAMED VEGGIES OR 1 CUP OF RICE	2 SLICES OF DELI TURKEY BREAST	TURKEY MEAT BALLS SERVED OVER 1 CUP OF SPAGHETTI SQUASH WITH LIGHT SAUCE

MEAL #1	SNACK	MEAL #2	SNACK	MEAL # 3
DAY 29 1/2 CUP OATMEAL WITH MIXED FRUIT,1 BOILED EGG	1 RICE CAKE WITH 2 TBSP OF LOW FAT PEANUT BUTTER	8 OZ BAKED COD FISH WITH 1 CUP OF STEAMED VEGGIES	1/2 CUP OF GREEK YOGURT AND 1/4 CUP OF FRIUT	8 OZ BBQ CHICKEN BREAST, 1 CUP STEAMED BROCCOLI
DAY 30 1 CUP OF FIBER CEREAL 1 SCOOP OF ISO-PROTEIN WITH 1/2 CUP OF FRUIT	1/2 AVOCADO WITH 1 TURKEY JERKEY	3 LEAN TURKEY MEAT BALLS SERVED OVER 1 CUP OF SPAGHETTI SQUASH WITH LIGHT SAUCE	1/2 GRAPFRUIT 1 TURKEY JERKEY	8 OZ BAKED WHITE FISH WITH 1 CUP OF STEAMED GREENS

30 DAY

SAMPLE MEAL PLAN COMPLETE

"NOTHING CAN STOP THE MAN WITH THE RIGHT MENTAL ATTITUDE FROM ACHIEVING HIS GOAL; NOTHING ON EARTH CAN HELP THE MAN WITH THE WRONG MENTAL ATTITUDE."

-THOMAS JEFFERSON

"NINETY-NINE PERCENT OF THE FAILURES COME FROM PEOPLE WHO HAVE THE HABIT OF MAKING EXCUSES."

-GEORGE WASHINGTON

CARVERR

IV WEEK QUICK BURST SPEED

WEEK I	WEEK II	WEEK III	WEEK IV
5X15 YD SPRINTS	5X15 YD SPRINTS	5X30 YD SPRINT	3X50 YD SPRINTS
3X20 YD SPRINTS	3X30 YD SPRINTS	3X15 YD SPRINTS	5X30 YD SPRINTS
1X50 YD SPRINTS	2X50 YD SPRINTS	5X10 YD SPRINTS	10X10 YD SPRINTS

*ADDITIONAL VI WEEK QUICK SPEED SPRINT PROGRAM CAN REPLACE OR BE ADDED TO YOUR ATHLETIC CROSS TRAINING PROGRAM. THIS SPEED PROGRAM WILL BE EFFECTIVE IN INCREASING A ATHLETES SPEED WHEN DONE A LEAST 3 DAYS A WEEK. RECOMMENDED PERCENT EFFORT IS AT 95-100% DUE TO SHORT BURST SPRINTS WITH 30-45 SECOND REST AND 1:00 -1:30 SECOND REST FOR LONGER SPRINTS.

ABOUT THE AUTHOR

Jacob Howell is an Award Winning Fitness Trainer and Strength Coach who has been recognized for his work with high school, college, and professional athletes for the past over 15 years. A former member of the St. Louis Cardinals organization strength staff and has a Natural World Fitness champion, Howell believes in hard work. His passion in helping athletes bring out the best in them through tough work and training is what motivates him. As a Texas high school coach well known for helping his athletes to develop in speed, strength, and total athletic performance, he brings innovative techniques; especially to under privileged athletes in South Texas. Howell has helped many high school athletes achieve their dreams to become collegiate athletes.

Howell holds a Master's degree of Science in Kinesiology and Health Education with emphasis in Human Performance from the University of Texas Pan American. He is a certified Strength and Conditioning Coach through the CSCCa completed at the University of Texas Austin. He has studied and worked under legendary Strength and Conditioning coaches Todd Stroud and Jon Jost at Florida State university, both former Strength Coaches of the Year, Coach D. Maib and Jeff "Maddog" Madden at the University of Texas Austin and President of CSCCa.

BIO:

Elite Nike SPARQ Trainer
B.S. & Master's Degree, CPT, SCCC - CSCCa
Over twelve years experience including high school, UT Austin, Florida State, St. Louis Cardinals
Certified College and Professional Strength & Conditioning Coach
Certified Speed Coach
Certified Personal Trainer
Donna ISD
PSJA ISD (North High School)
Mercedes ISD
Concordia University Austin TX.
Private tactical , strength & Condition trainer for Police and Military clients

Contact Info (863) 458 6300

www.ingramcontent.com/pod-product-compliance
Lightning Source LLC
Chambersburg PA
CBHW062050280526
45788CB00003B/1178